I0838885

THE REFLECTION OF MY *soul*

Secrets of a story of self-healing

Natalia Orsi

This book is a testimony, and it reflects the personal experience of the author. It should not be interpreted as a guide to self-healing. If you intend to follow any of the book's exercises or suggestions, do so solely under the supervision of a physician or a healthcare professional.

ISBN: 9798729361069
Edition: Natalia Orsi
Graphic Design: Andrés Torrents
Translation: Mariana Amestoy
Original title of this book: *El reflejo de mi alma.*
1st edition: Abril 2021
For more information visit:
www.elreflejodemialma.com

"Miracles are not contrary to nature, but only contrary to what we know about nature."

Saint Augustine.

DEDICATION

This book is dedicated to all those on the path of physical, mental, and spiritual healing.

Note to English Translation
To Natalia's Readers from Yana M.

Lost in translation…

If you've ever tried to learn any new language, then you may have
come to the conclusion that translating is not always an easy affair.
For all of you multilingual speakers you have certainly come across the
perfect word in one language to express a particular situation, concept
or feeling, and would be hard-pressed to find one word to convey the
same meaning in another language. One usually resorts to a someti-
mes-lengthy explanation to convey all that is associated with a simple
word.

Having had the honor to be involved and to have read Natalia's book
" The Reflection of my Soul" from inception to completion in its original
Spanish version, I would like to add a few notes to amplify nuances and
meanings that may not have been conveyed in the English version.

Natalia does a great job drawing you into her healing journey and into
her world. She does use throughout her writing the diminutive Spanish
suffixes: "ito" and "ita", which is a great way for a Spanish speaker to
convey an endearing and affectionate quality to that particular word,
thus situation.

I've compiled a list of a few that are sprinkled throughout her story
so that you would appreciate the depth of Natalia's connection with
what is important to her. She uses them profusely when describing
her grandmothers, family, nature and anything related to her home
town. These words in the diminutive form become a gate, a doorway
to Natalia's heart, to her magical world, which then held the power of
her self-healing.

From the bottom of my heart, I hope that as you read these endearing
words throughout her story, you'll keep in mind the importance they've
held in Natalia's world, and how somehow, they became the key to
unlocking her connection to her own divine power.

May these words unlock your own divine healing powers!

Diminutive words that couldn't be translated:

Diminutive form (Non Diminutive Word in Spanish: "Little" Translation)

Feminine Words "ita" :

Abuelita (Abuela: "Little" grand mother)
Bajita (Baja : "Little" short in size)
Chiquita (Chica: "Little" small)
Flaquita (Flaca : "Little" skinny)
Lucecita (Luz : "Small, Little" light)
Carita (Cara: "Little" face) (As when she mentions Smiley Faces and God….read on….)
Ollita (Olla: "Little" Pan)
Escuelita (Escuela: "Little" School)
Vecinita (Vecina: "Little" Neighbor)
Princecita (Princesa: "Little" Princess
Florecita (Flor: "Little" Flower)
Semillita (Semilla: "Little" Seed)
Lamparita de luz (Lampara: "Little" Lamp)
Cambiadita (Cambiar – changed : as in appearance/ clothes)

Masculine Words "ito" :

Papelito (Papel : "Little" Paper)
Perfumito (Perfume: "Little" Perfume)
Huevitos (Huevo: "Little" Eggs)
Animalitos (Animal: "Little" Animals)
Bichito (Bicho: "Little" Critter, Bug)
Tecito (Te: "Little" Tea) (when referring to her medicinal tea o tea time with grand mother)
Tecito calentito (Te Caliente: "Little" Hot Tea)
Pastorcitos (Pastor: "Little" Shepards) (When she mention Virgen Mary of Fatima Portugal)
Rinconcito (Rincon: "Little" Corner)
Elefantito (Elefante: "Little" Elephant)
Angelito (Angel: "Little" Angel)
Sapito (Sapo: "Little" Toad) (As when she mentions... fear of toads)
Regalitos (Regalo: "Little" Presents)

The following show compassion towards herself and others:

Pasito (Paso: "Little" Step)
Despacito (Despacio: "Little" Slow(er))
Empujoncito (Empujon: "Little" Push)

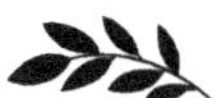

CONTENTS

Introduction

Soul on fire — 23

The place I chose to be born — 33

My refuge: resistance — 41

Song of angels — 49

An unwavering promise — 55

My enchanted garden under lock and key — 61

The last call — 69

God's daughter — 77

My life's teacher — 83

Divine guidance towards the magic potion — 89

The reflection of my soul — 99

Between heaven and earth — 107

Sacred treasure — 113

You are unique, and you have an agreement with God — 133

Special: May your body be a sanctuary! — 137

Acknowledgments

Glossary

Bibliography

About the author

INTRODUCTION

Thank you for holding me in your hands, with a desire to know my story and the hope to heal, much alive.

The universe is ready to help us. We create by attracting what is necessary for us at every given moment. With this intention in mind, I would like to sow a seed of trust, a seed of self confidence, for you to understand that you are not alone, that what happens to you and what you do is as perfect and necessary as you.

We all have our life story, so personal, so unique, and so close to us.

The story we have lived throughout the years is the ideal setting to carry out our purpose, the awakening of our consciousness, the path towards healing our soul, and our human nature.

Without you, it wouldn't be the same.

We are part of a divine plan that relies on us, waits for us, pushes and encourages us, and, we can feel it by observing and loving ourselves, in every beat of our heart.

It is my desire that the most hidden secrets of this story of love, forgiveness, and healing awaken within you.

I am here, willing to lend you a hand and hold you tight with an open heart, because, if we are not living in this world to help each other, our existence would not make any sense.

Multiple sclerosis was the disease that manifested in my physical body to get my attention. It pulled the emergency brake on my life when I was about to crash.

The disease was my greatest blessing, my noble friend, the one who made me fight with myself until I lost all strength. It came to ask me questions and more questions, for which I had no answers.

It forced me to look for alternatives, to get out of my comfort zone, and to undo who I thought I was.

It faithfully stayed with me until it completed its mission: to leave me standing on the path towards the healing of my soul.

I have devoted the past few years of my life understanding what happened, the reason I reached a state of illness, and healing itself.

All the existential questions that had been there since I was a child resurfaced. I knew that if I came to understand our existence, life itself, I would understand the reason for my illness and the miracle of healing.

We can look at life in many ways. Each of us has a theory of what we think life is, which may or may not change depending on our life experiences.

Looking at life has always been a part of me. I have observed it, questioned it, challenged it, investigated it, and respected it.

My greatest passion has always been to discover the secrets that lie behind life.

Life in itself has been my constant motivation.

Healing a disease that, for now, "has no cure" was definitely one of the most beautiful challenges of my life. It has been a long and amazing journey, hand in hand with divine guidance which led me to unimaginable places and beings, and to my childhood back and forth nonstop. It made me realize what it is to feel, and to be amazed, time after time, and say, "I can't believe it"! while an inner voice would tell me: "yes, it is so!."

And so, I continued, I questioned everything, verified what I could, always stood behind my doubts, asked for clarity, signs, and life itself brought me the answers in many different ways.

I learned to listen, wait, see, accept, forgive, feel, heal, and even smile at the hardest things I experienced.

So many mysteries to be discovered! It was time to see reality from a fresh perspective and open my mind and heart like never before.

Here I would like to share with you my healing experience from multiple sclerosis, reconstructed and integrated, and presented in these pages through the most sacred paths of the heart.

Enjoy it!

"

*If nothing existed beyond this world, if nothing existed beyond this life, if there were no purpose to which we were all committed, my life would have no meaning.***"**

A SOUL ON FIRE

I could say the pain I felt that day in my body and soul was so intense that my crying was heard in the heavens.

It was almost three in the afternoon in the city of Dubai. I was walking on the sidewalk of Jumeirah Beach Road on the way to an appointment I had made with an acupuncturist.

The asphalt was boiling with the desert heat. The sun's rays reflected on the vast white wall that ran along that block and on my red face full of tears.

I was walking, feeling broken in a state of despair and helplessness. I had been experiencing a burning sensation in my left leg for a few days now, and couldn't find any explanation for it. I didn't know what was happening to me.

I arrived at the acupuncturist's office, but he didn't inspire me with confidence. The pain from the needles was so acute that I kept crying uncontrollably and asked him to remove them. The burning sensation got worse, and I could feel it all over my body.

Back home, terrified of what could happen, all I knew was that I couldn't escape.

It was 2009, and my husband Alejandro and I had been living for nine months in the city of Dubai, in the United Arab Emirates.

The intention to start a new adventure was so strong that, after talking about it, and without giving it too much thought, a month later we were landing at the Dubai airport with our belongings, in sweltering heat and during the time of Ramadan*, something new that we learned about as soon as we set foot on Arab soil.

I can now see that the universe conspired so that with the desert as the backdrop we would live there the most remarkable experiences of our lives.

I called my mother in Casbas, my hometown in Argentina, to tell her how I felt and ask her to get in touch with our family doctor to let him know about my symptoms.

Frantic with worry, my mom called me back right away and asked me to have my blood pressure checked and to see a doctor as soon as possible.

The next day Alejandro and I finished work at noon and went to look for a hospital where I could have my blood pressure checked.

Back then, a construction boom overtook the city of Dubai. There were machines digging wells everywhere, cranes, trucks, workers, detour signs, and sand flying all around. The streets had no names and changed course every day, and there were no maps. We had never been to a hospital in Dubai, but we got there asking around.

At first, we went to the American Hospital which had been recommended to us, and it was close by, but only stayed for 5 minutes as nobody came to help us.

I needed care. I couldn't wait.

On the way to the beach side, we arrived at the Neuro Spinal Hospital emergency room on Jumeirah Beach Road.

We were not aware then that the Neuro Spinal Hospital, funded in 2002, was the first hospital in Dubai specializing in neuroscience.

While waiting in the emergency room, I kept receiving and sending work emails as if nothing happened. I was already getting used to the burning sensation and the pain in my leg.

They checked my blood pressure, my body temperature, and tested the knees' reflexes. The doctor prescribed an immediate magnetic resonance imaging of the brain.

It was the first time I had an MRI done. I remembered hearing that the confinement inside the machine was not a pleasant experience.

They moved me to a remote wing of the hospital; over there, the lights were dim, and it was very silent.

I took a deep breath. A specialist greeted me, gave me a gown, explained to me how the procedure would be, and told me that the exam would take approximately 45 minutes.

I left with the gown to the dressing room. I took my clothes off and placed them on a chair, covering my underwear with my shirt.

Holding the gown, I turned it around several times trying to figure out how I should wear it. I didn't know if the opening should go in the front or the back.

I decided that if they had to see me, they would see me from behind. I blushed.

I remember the gown, spotless clean, nicely ironed and a lovely smell, making you feel like they thought of you and wanted to take care of you... But that wasn't enough; I knew something was wrong, and I didn't know what it was.

What I felt there all by myself in that hospital dressing room is indescribable: there, you have no choice but to surrender to the hands of a specialist who will perform your procedure, and later on will hand over the results to the doctor, then he'll go home.

You'll never know who that person is, nor his name, nor will he divulge what he saw in your body, you only know that those images will be the backdrop for your new story to unfold; the images will be the only thing you'll take with you.

I walked into a large room, no windows, and I lay down with half of my body inside the MRI machine. Motionless.

The technician was operating the system from outside the room; a glass panel separated us, should I have screamed he would not have been able to hear me.

He gave me a remote control to send him a warning in case something happened, but if I did, he would have to interrupt the procedure and start all over again.

When the procedure started, I felt extremely anxious. I did some breathing exercises to calm myself down, but at times, I would feel the urge to ask the specialist to please let me out of there.

It was a constant battle with my mind. The machine's sound: tac, tac, tac; I couldn't tell what was going on. I thought: "Am I getting radiation? This may damage my brain", so I kept trying to focus on something else. I would visualize being on a river, at sea, on a mountain, planning what I would do after leaving the hospital, what we would have for dinner. Then, other thoughts would flood my mind, such as "Is the tecnician still there? He wouldn't leave, right?"

Such suffering!

Once the procedure ended, we had to wait for the results in another room.

The doctor came in with a concerned look on his face. The results were not encouraging, as they had suspected from the beginning. It looked as if I had experienced a stroke.

At that very moment, making direct eye contact, the doctor said: "You need to be hospitalized."

With the phone in one hand, my purse over my shoulder, and Alejandro by my side, there was a moment of silence when I thought: "How strange! My head feels fine. I've never felt anything strange." But I instinctively agreed. I accepted; certainly with the current outlook I wasn't going anywhere.

And so it was; I was hospitalized for ten days at the Neuro Spinal Hospital of Dubai.

During that time, many things happened. Alejandro and I were young and found ourselves alone in a distant foreign country, in a hospital room, without understanding much what was happening to my health.

The doctors were Iraqi. They would come early in the morning to my room; a team of three, they always came in together. They would stand and look at me from the foot of the bed. They spoke in Arabic, and they would leave without saying a word.

I had many tests and medical studies done during that time: blood and urine, a lumbar puncture to extract a cerebrospinal fluid sample, and MRIs with and without contrast.

With contrast a fluid is used to greatly enhance the image quality. They would inject the fluid while I would lie inside the MRI scanner; I felt a burning sensation like lightening passing through my brain.

By now, my entire body had been inside these scanners several times. I got them to play some background music in the room, where I spent two hours, while they performed MRIs of my brain and spinal cord.

My arms had no room left to insert one more needle.

Back then, they would send the tests to Germany since there was no specialized laboratory in Dubai.

In the meantime, I kept feeling the burning sensation in my leg, but I was more relaxed. From the window, I could see Jumeirah Beach and the palm trees, but I didn't feel like taking a walk. It was scorching hot, and I would rather lie down and have them take care of me.

Many friends came to visit me at the hospital, bringing delicious food from our home country and fashion magazines to distract me. Coworkers also came over bearing gifts.

One day Tushar, a coworker from India, came to see me with a basket full of fruits; I remember the only thing he said with a smile was: "mam*, you have to eat more fruits."

He was a person of few words, but he would smile. I thanked him for his gift. Then as I looked at him I realized that he had been observing me, and there he was, with his message at the perfect time.

Those days at the hospital were a break from my hectic life, a much-needed rest, that for too long, I had not allowed myself to take.

Regardless of my health diagnosis, I felt looked after and cared for; my body was resting. I didn't want to think about anything; my mind was blank as if I had entrusted those doctors with my health condition, without expectations or thoughts, either negative or positive. I didn't draw any conclusions either.

My state of mind had reached a limit such that I had no strength left to process information.

Several days went by, and no one would tell us anything about what was going on. We knew it would take a long time to get the test results back from Germany but came a point when knowing a bit more would have put us all at ease. Though truthfully somehow at that particular point it was the same to me, to know or not to know.

Alejandro convinced the doctors to come over to see me on a Saturday morning.

Two of them came into the room, crossed arms and one hand under their chin, looking quite concerned; the older one, the hospital director, looked at me and calmly said: "you have multiple sclerosis."

Lying down on the bed, I asked: "What is multiple sclerosis?" as if they were not talking about me. And the doctor answered: "it is a disease which, for the time being, has no cure, but we can control it …". At that point, I stopped listening; I told myself: "whatever multiple sclerosis is, what they are telling me is not happening to me."

Over the next five days, they gave me several intravenous doses of corticosteroid to suppress the inflammation of the nervous tissues.

Corticosteroids mimic a natural hormone produced by the adrenal glands. They replace that hormone when our bodies don't make enough of it.

In a matter of minutes, that dose would make the symptom disappear. The symptom I was having was a burning sensation in my leg. With the first dose, the burning sensation disappeared altogether.

The doctors recommended a drug treatment that could keep the illness from progressing.

They said that this treatment is for life. They handed me a piece of paper with the names of all the drugs available on the market so that I would choose which one to try first since, depending on the patient, some drugs work and others do not.

I kept the paper in my purse without looking at it.

They discharged me, telling me I had to keep taking the corticosteroid pills at home for another ten days.

I left the hospital as if there was nothing wrong with me.

When I finished the corticosteroids, my face remained swollen for a while, but I had no symptoms. Without thinking about anything or anyone and without being asked to, I returned to work and resumed my everyday life.

THE PLACE I CHOSE TO BE BORN

I was born and lived in the province of Buenos Aires, Argentina, until my adolescence. I always say I had a happy childhood in the countryside, although we lived some blocks away from the actual countryside.

My dad was a farmer, and my mother was a teacher at a rural school. I have a sister and a brother; I am the oldest of the three. We're a dynamic and unique family, connected and fond of nature, of beauty, of the simple things of life, and above all, of freedom.

During my childhood, we spent a great deal of time at our grandmothers' homes.

My maternal grandmother's name was Lucía; we called her "grandmother Lucía"; she was the daughter of Portuguese immigrants.

Of my great grandparents, I only met my great grandmother; her name was Felicidad. She lived with one of her children, "uncle" Manuel; her house was next to grandmother Lucía and my grandmother's other brother, "uncle" José.

Behind their houses there were only fruit orchards and vegetable gardens, overflowing with fruits and vegetables of all sorts and variety. We could cross from one orchard to the other as chicken would run about free.

They lived in different houses, but sharing the bountiful, always spending time together.

They taught me about the rhythms of nature, the labor to get its fruits,

its natural pharmacy, and above everything else, how to be of service to others.

From outside, as we would approach my great-grandmother's house, we could sniff the smell of boiling vegetables for the soup. Juana, the lady who looked after her, would make the most delicious soups I have ever had.

I remember my 90-year-old great-grandmother lying down on her bed during nap time ("siesta"). My grandmother Lucía would always keep her company with a loving smile. She would bathe her, comb her hair, and sprinkle powder and her favorite perfume on her skin. I loved to be there with them, to bring to my grandmother whatever she needed for her to enjoy seeing her mother joyfully singing in her cherished Portuguese, and waiting, all dressed up, for some guest to show up for "mate*" time.

My grandmother Lucía used to tell me that my great-grandmother Felicidad had always missed her homeland, Portugal. She did not like Argentina; she came with her boyfriend, my great-grandfather Francisco, looking for a job during wartime; they started a family, and they did well. However, it was painful for her; she could have gone back to visit Portugal, but she preferred not to. She didn't want to go through another goodbye. Now and then, she would send a letter and get an answer, but that was it.

We would spend the afternoon hours drinking mate in silence, looking at the sunset out the window. Sometimes we would share memories and delightful anecdotes for upcoming birthdays or anniversaries, or talk a bit about the weather. And while the mate was passed around from one to another, I would get excited rummaging through the furniture drawers filled with stories, unique scents, and maybe looking for my ancestor's life experiences that could define me.

I recall in one room in my great-grandmother's house, there was a huge box with stuff left by a young cousin of my mother who was studying in Buenos Aires.

In that box, there were cardstock papers, handmade drawings, colored pencils, hats, Snoopy pins, books by different authors: it was like a box full of surprises. What I remember the most was a card with the words "God is Love" along with a smiley face.

At the time I thought it was "cool" to write "God is love" and draw smiley faces around it since my mother's cousin seemed like a "cool" person to me. She was studying far away, and every time she came back, she would bring news from the city. The fact that she kept the card meant something to me.

That image I shall forever remember, and I knew it had great significance. Back then, I didn't fully understand it.

Grandmother Lucía was very active, attentive to her appearance, slender with green eyes. She would always attend to all of us, visit the sick and old friends, bring presents, and share the fruits and vegetables from her garden with her neighbors.

She was the one who taught us that pinching and pulling the skin of someone's back heals a stomachache, that linden tea calms us down, that breathing medicinal bay leaves from a pot with boiling water heals a cold, and hot cotton pads on the chest relieves coughs. She would also say that we could cure indigestion at a distance, that hot water bottles were a loving treat for our feet on chilly nights, that taking a nap gives us energy for the second half of the day, that flowers smile at us, and that sweeping the sidewalk, when done with love, will fill us with inner peace.

Grandmother Lucía would welcome anyone from the town who would knock at the door looking for work. There was always someone busy with varied chores: sweeping the patio, picking up fruits that fell to the ground, painting a wall, or fixing wires in the chicken coop. She would always find something so those who were seeking a job could work and buy food that day. She would welcome them as she would any other guest, with a glass of water, some mate, a piece of bread, or coffee with milk [café con leche]. She would chat, listen to them, and welcome them to sit with us to share an afternoon snack.

Because of that, we met many beautiful people and learned many stories.

She was also the one who would let us win when playing cards, would take us to all the funerals in town, would let us wear her clothes and jewelry to go out on the streets all dressed up; she passed onto us her fear of toads, and she would invite us to enjoy tea or "mate" with cake, pastries, or "buñuelos "[fritters] that she would make to entertain her friends.

Her days would brighten by being of service...that's what her life was all about.

My paternal grandmother, Marina, came from a family of Italian immigrants. She had many similarities with my grandmother Lucía and also something extraordinary: she loved, with her whole being, God.

She saw God in everything: the snails in the garden, the pigeons of the pigeon loft, the ants that ate the stale bread from her pantry, and in the roses of her garden. She looked at everything with tenderness, and talked to them with conviction: "snail, come here! Leave that lettuce alone!", "ant, you are hungry, come so that I can feed you out here, don't go into my pantry"; those moments when she, the ant, and I were there, or when she, the snail, the lettuce, and I were there seemed like a fairy tale. Magical moments.

She was short and hunchbacked, so much so that she could touch the floor with her hands. Sometimes she would ask us to help her stand up straight; with some pain, she would manage to do so, and wherever we went, we would take her by the arm.

We took turns among my cousins to keep her company at night; if you were older than six, then you could stay with grandmother. But for sure, you had to be willing to have an early dinner, take a bath with a small pot of hot water, go to bed early, pray next to her and get up at sunrise.

At dawn, she would lift the blinds, the sunlight would hit your face, and you would hear: "come on, darling, let's get up."

Hers were love stories, about her boyfriend, grandfather Armando, about their life together, about her brothers and sisters, about how important it was to do things right; I remember her telling me: "life is beautiful, darling."

Her days would brighten by seeing God through nature... That was her life.

During all those happy years, there was also someone very much present and important to me: God, mine only, but back then, I didn't call Him that; He didn't have a name.

Deep within me, I have the memory that God asked me to be born on Earth to help Him with a task and that I accepted; I have images of that moment in Heaven before coming here. It may have been a dream, or someone may have told me about it, or maybe it is so, and the memory lives in my heart.

With Him, I had a sense of eternal love, infinite connection, unbreakable friendship, absolute protection, and mystery. He came with me everywhere. He was my God, or however you choose to call it: divine energy, the universe itself— that "something" which is much greater than all of us.

And that's how I grew up, loving nature and my family, enjoying a new adventure every day, hand in hand with an energy from beyond.

During my childhood, I had many questions I did not dare to ask, perhaps because I thought people would not understand me.

Once there were many people at my home, all of them sitting around the table having lunch, and all speaking at the same time—the Italian way. From the outside looking in, you couldn't follow a conversation.

I was eight years old at the time, and I remember, as if it were today, that while I was looking at all of them, a sense of distrust came over me, and I asked myself: What is all this? What are we doing here? Why are they sitting around a table? What does this all mean? I walked behind them and grabbed them by the neck, one by one as if attempting to remove a mask. I thought they might be wearing costumes and acting so that I would believe the fiction. I don't really know, but it surprised me to find out it wasn't the case, that their heads were in fact, attached to their bodies.

I don't think anyone noticed. Some of them looked at me without looking at me; maybe something annoyed them, but nobody asked me anything; they were all in their own world.

There were other instances like that one. Somehow, I was always wondering whether we were real.

I couldn't understand the fact that each one had a role: my dad, my mom, my siblings, I, who was the oldest daughter, that my relatives were specific individuals and not others, that there were rules for eating, getting dressed, prearranged activities, that I had to go to school, and follow schedules for everything, that there were seven days of the week, that we had to sleep through the night, that we have dreams... Why were my neighbors my neighbors, and not my siblings? How was everything determined? Who decided everything?

I didn't understand the meaning of a lot of things, even so I adapted to everything.

MY REFUGE:
RESISTANCE

I kept living a normal life. I couldn't believe that I was sick with multiple sclerosis. Where did the disease come from?

How could something like this happen to me? It was impossible; I had always been very healthy. I grew up eating fruits and vegetables from the garden, had never been sick, and never took medications nor drugs. At home, we used herbal teas or Bach flowers as medicine. I lived a calm life; I had no sleeping problems; I was athletic, had friends everywhere, a job, and I would travel...

The memories of drinking alcohol during outings when I lived in Miami started coming to my mind... mixtures from any bottle, but not more than other single person that goes out to dance and have fun.

Of course, I looked for culprits: who could I blame for what happened to me? But I would also wonder if there could actually be a culprit... The cause of multiple sclerosis, to this day, is unknown, although the suspected cause is a virus or a novel antigen. They also believe it can be genetic.

When I read it could be a virus, I laughed. I couldn't wrap my mind around the fact that a virus would affect a few people scattered around the world: I didn't know anyone who had been around me during the past few years who had that disease...if it was a virus, it should be contagious.

"Could it be that it affects those of us with a specific DNA? That made more sense to me, but how could I find out?"

It could be genetic. I asked my family but no one knew of anyone who had multiple sclerosis nor any of the symptoms that occur with this disease. Perhaps some relatives had it and never found out. It was still unclear to me.

I didn't recognize myself.

Jacqueline, an American coworker, 60 years old, very tall, blonde with straight hair, wore glasses, and loved fire trucks. Her dream was to return to the United States and buy a few of them. She used to say that there were many fires where she came from, so that fire trucks would be her best investment.

One afternoon we had to visit a client, so we took a taxicab together.

We took Sheikh Zayed Road, a multilane road, almost a highway that runs through Dubai from beginning to end. As we passed by the old area where the first buildings were located, before arriving at Al Safa*, she told me: "Nati, look up there... the buildings, how beautiful!"

In her voice, there was gratitude to life in itself for allowing her to enjoy such an extraordinary view.

I thought: "What does she see in those buildings? They are in the middle of the desert. They are all brown, covered with dirt and dust; there isn't a place uglier than this. Where does she see the beauty?

So as not to ruin the moment, I replied, "yeah, they're amazing!"

When we are ill, we lose pleasure in things. Nothing wonders us anymore, we shut down, and we cannot see the beauty in anything or anyone. The problem is that we are not even aware of it.

Back then, I met some people with multiple sclerosis. I remember a British woman who worked on the fourth floor of the building where I worked. She had to have a drug injected into her belly every single day for the past seven years.

Once she showed me her belly, she looked at me and said: "this doesn't have a cure; this is for life. What's more, the medication is very expensive."

I had heard that Majid Al Futtaim*, the company owner where we worked, helped her buy the medication. I wondered what this woman was going to do when she didn't work there anymore.

The thought that I would also receive help to pay for the medication briefly crossed my mind... How could that medication be so expensive if it didn't even cure you?

It was a terrifying perspective; somehow, I turned a deaf ear; I had never envisioned that kind of future, and I would not do so now.

The time had come when society considered me seriously ill.

It was very unusual for somebody to mention anything about my disease. I am not sure if people didn't dare to or if I didn't give them the space to do it.

I always remember the father of a friend of mine who came to Dubai to visit. We were outside in her garden; there were many people. They were barbecuing, and there was music; everybody was talking. We were both sitting outside. He reminded me a lot of my father: his age, his history, his way of speaking. It was pleasant to talk to him.

At one point, he told me: "my daughter mentioned to me something about what the doctors told you." He paused.

I replied with a shaky voice: "yes, they diagnosed me with multiple sclerosis." He stared at me and responded only with a gesture to let me know he was very sorry. I smiled at him.

We remained silent.

At that very moment, I remembered my parents, and I felt their concern and silence, the same silence conveyed by my friend's father.

I felt the grief of what this reality meant to them.

I felt their worry and fear around me. Every day I give thanks for not paying attention to people's comments, such as "maybe you should"; neither did I allow what people wanted to tell me to interfere with my state of mind and actions. I knew this issue was mine and only mine. No one else knew how I felt and what I needed.

What I needed the most was not to believe that I was sick. I was at the point of processing the entire picture. I needed space, silence, and to continue with the life I had, which, except for my health, was not bad.

I couldn't look at reality and accept that I was sick. I knew that if I did, people would convince me to take medications, and I didn't want that for myself.

If I declared myself ill, there would be no chance that I or someone else could help me.

Resistance to everything was my refuge. I didn't let my mind wander through places where I did not want it to go. I was afraid to lose control of my life, of what I was, and to give it to someone who did not understand what this change meant to me.

And I did just that. I didn't listen to anyone; I waited to see what would happen, still carrying the burden of the disease on my shoulders.

Today I know that there was a soul by my side at all times who knew how to support me... Alejandro.

He was there to listen to me and respect my moments of silence.

He had great faith in me and in whatever was meant to happen.

SONG OF
ANGELS

A few months after going through the first episode of multiple sclerosis, I arrived at work one day at around eight in the morning and looked for a place in the Deira City Centre parking lot, a shopping mall in front of the building.

I was happy. It was a beautiful day; I was wearing new clothes that I had bought to go to work.

I parked my car in an empty spot. And suddenly, an explosion! I slowly tried to open my eyes. It felt as if I had fainted. I found myself covered with dust, which was stuck everywhere: the airbag had exploded!

When I tried to open the door, I could not move my left arm: the airbag's impact fractured both of my forearm bones, the radius, and the ulna, in two parts.

I felt the pain of the arm as it was hanging, so I tried to fix it with my other hand, placing it on my chest. I tried to open the door with my right hand and screamed: Help! Help! Someone who worked in my building saw me and came running, called the police, the ambulance, and Alejandro.

The police couldn't understand how everything happened: my car was parked, and there were no scratches on the front. Somehow, the vehicle touched the low wall in front of it, causing the airbag to activate. To this day, what happened remains a mystery.

The only thing I remember after being taken into the ambulance is that I asked them to slow down. Whenever the ambulance would make a sudden movement, brake, turn or speed up, my arm would move, and the pain was unbearable.

We arrived at Rashid Hospital, a very important general medicine and surgery hospital in Dubai. After being admitted, they took X-rays.

They left me in a room, sitting on a stretcher, waiting until I could have surgery. I had fractured and splintered my bones.

There I was, at the hospital, in absolute agony.

The pain was so excruciating that I no longer felt it. A cry of pain came out from deep within me as if coming from my soul. I always say dogs make the same sound when they cry or are sad or injured.

We waited for ten hours to have surgery.

As I entered the room where they prepare patients for surgery, I told the doctors that I had multiple sclerosis (it was hard for me to utter those words!). Still, I did, in case the general anesthesia could be a problem ... I also told them I could be pregnant.

They did a pregnancy test right there, and sure enough, it came back positive. The nurses and anesthesiologists all congratulated me... I couldn't believe it. What a strange situation!

Lying on a stretcher on the way to the operating room. We passed by Alejandro and a couple who were friends of ours. She was from Spain, and he was French. And I was screaming: I am pregnant!!!

The surgery went very well. They used a metal plate to join the bones, and with so many stitches, my arm looked like "matambre cocido" [stuffed and stitched rolled beef, a typical Argentine meat dish].

That evening after the surgery, they took me to the women's ward of the hospital. There was no private room available at the moment.

In the Arab world, it's important to separate men from women. They design everything so that men and women do not cross paths.

Therefore, Alejandro could not visit me in the room.

I spent two nights at the hospital.

I remember that a friend I met in Dubai, from Guaminí (a town 30 kilometers away from mine in Argentina), came to visit me at the hospital with a vegetable tart that she made to enjoy together; and the mate! And so, behind the curtains around my hospital bed, we traveled back to our beloved land.

The nights in that hospital room were quiet. Luckily, I was close to the nurses' area, most of them from the Philippines. They chatted and laughed all night long. They were very friendly!

What stands out the most from my experience at Rashid Hospital was a grandmother on a bed diagonally across from mine. She was very short, petite, and skinny, and her hair was all white.

Every night, sitting on the bed, she would put on her nightgown, comb her hair, and puff talcum powder on her face, neck, and hands. She would lie down, cover herself, and sing to her God. Allah! Allah! Allah! Allah*! were the lyrics of her melody. It was the only sound we heard in the room. All of us there, over ten women and the nurses, would listen quietly to her voice, so beautiful, so precious.

In the mornings, from early on, she would be ready, changed, and perfumed. As soon as they announced that her son was waiting for her, she would walk out slowly to greet him in the visitor's room.

When I remember those days, I daydream and imagine that the lady was the Arab version of my great-grandmother Felicidad, that she had come to that hospital room to let me know: she was there with me, by my side, with her stories, her memories, her white hair, the fragrance of the talcum powder, and her song of angels.

That grandmother was a light, a messenger; she was faith and gratitude.

On the other hand, looking at my arm full of stitches and with no mobility, I knew what was ahead: two months of rehabilitation at home, without being able to go to work.

The universe conspired once again to slow down my pace, so that I would stop, and see that there were other priorities I was not taking care of. There was something much more important, and I was not paying attention to it.

AN UNWAVERING PROMISE

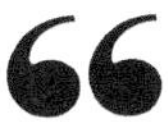

After the accident, I enjoyed my pregnancy as I never thought I would. I took the time to learn how to become a mom, and buy everything I needed for the baby, and prepare for her arrival with much love. It was wonderful.

Besides, I was happier because nature's wisdom makes multiple sclerosis dormant during pregnancy.

I remember the doctor telling me that perhaps I should have many children; that made me laugh.

But the disease took it upon itself to remind me it was still there. After delivering my daughter, my body's natural defenses dropped, and I had a new episode. It happened a month after my daughter Catalina was born.

Little by little, my feet became numb. Within a couple of days, my hands and feet were intensely tingling.

My parents were visiting us in Dubai. I decided to go to the hospital as the tingling worsened, and I knew it would not stop.

The hospital admitted me right away, and they did all the necessary checkups, tests, and MRI procedures.

After waiting for the results, they called us into the doctor's office, one of the original Iraqi physicians. I was there with my husband and my dad.

The room was chilly and dark. I remember there were pictures of human bodies hanging everywhere on the white walls. I was looking at the pictures; we were all silent while the doctor opened his computer.

There was no doubt about it: I had new lesions in the brain and spinal cord. The doctor showed us every image and described each detail. He talked to me a lot. He asked me to please consider to start taking the drugs, to understand that there was no cure for multiple sclerosis and that the drugs could control the disease so that it wouldn't progress.

My husband asked me to think about it, and my father, to whom we had been translating what the doctor was saying, told me: "Nati, what are you going to do? Perhaps it's for the best, you have the baby now; well, I don't know what to tell you."

With the list of all the drugs available on the market, which once again the doctor wrote on a piece of paper for me to take home, and his message of hope that the treatment might help control the progress of the disease, I found the courage to say to all three: "Give me another chance, this is the last one, I promise!"

The silence, acceptance, and respect that I felt from these three amazing beings was undoubtedly the first step towards my healing.

"If I became sick on my own, I should be able to heal on my own."

"I brought the disease, and now I have to let it go."

"The human body is so perfect that it must have a way, a mechanism to regenerate and heal."

"I don't believe that God designed our bodies to be able to get sick without being able to heal."

Those were my thoughts.

I didn't speak with anyone about my thoughts. I had declared to myself long ago that this challenge was mine alone. I knew that asking for opinions would delay my healing.

I devoted myself to become a mom and enjoy my parents, who stayed with us for several months.

Later on, we traveled to my home country, Argentina, to enjoy the summer there with our daughter. I spent Christmas at my parents' house with my family and siblings, and the New Year at the beach in Uruguay, with my brothers- and sisters-in-law, nieces and nephews.

Everything was fine when I was away from the Neuro Spinal Hospital. I didn't think at all about the issue. I blocked it.

The promise I made was so powerful that I thought it would have benefits on its own, and by being far away from the Neuro Spinal Hospital, I assumed that the disease was not with me, that it had stayed in Dubai, perhaps with my doctor.

From the other side of the world, whenever I thought about my Iraqi doctor, the hospital, the nurses, and the MRI, I saw everything very differently.

It was an image foreign to me, a sad, cold, depressing, and hopeless one.

At that particular moment, I was on vacation with my family, what I loved most in the world, so I didn´t want to be disturbed with that issue.

MY ENCHANTED GARDEN
UNDER LOCK AND KEY

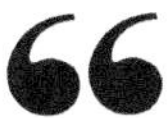

For a few years, my sister and I attended a rural school at Casey, an abandoned old railroad station. The school was in the middle of the countryside.

Teachers from all the nearby towns would go to teach the children who lived in the surrounding farms and rural areas.

My mom was one of those teachers.

Casey's old school, where my grandmother Lucía and her siblings studied, was behind our school.

It was an enchanted, abandoned place, surrounded by trees and medicinal laurel. Half of the walls had crumbled and from underneath the rubble flowers and lovegrass would grow.

It was so special to spend my days as a child playing in that school, knowing that, as children, my grandmother and siblings played on that same floor, in that same place, at the old school behind.

Sometimes, I would imagine them running around during recess, and I would think how wonderful it would be to go back in time and be able to see them.

My classmates and friends came to school on horseback, tractor, or in the back of pick up trucks. They were always happy, dressed in white smocks, and wore their hair in a bun or combed with hair gel.

They lived very connected to nature, and knew everything about animals: their reproduction, hiding places, and qualities. Whenever we found small eggs hidden under a tree or in the bushes, they knew if they came from a chicken, a duck, a goose, an ostrich, or a snake.

I remember they would say: "This is the time when barn swallows migrate!", and the day would come when we would see the flocks of barn swallows from the school playground across the blue sky in the springtime.

I remember trying to picture their lives and wonder: "What do they think about my sister and me? They showed much respect towards us; sometimes they seemed embarrassed to talk to us, perhaps because we were from the nearby town and we were the teacher's daughters.

I had a friend who would always play with me: she had three sisters; they were all very close, and they always seemed very happy.

One day we invited her to my house for lunch after school. Her family had to go shopping in town that afternoon, so they would pick her up later from my home.

We had a lot of fun while having lunch. She seemed excited; my mom had bought a dessert with bananas and "dulce de leche" for us. I will never forget when she asked: "Can I eat a whole banana all by myself? And we responded yes, with a smile.

Back then, I was eight years old, and in the country school, I saw a different way of life with different values and possibilities, but this was the first time I had experienced it so closely.

We also had friends in the city. When we were at my grandmother's house, some neighbors came to play with us. We called them: "the friends from grandmother's house."

One of them always wanted to go inside the kitchen to wash the juice glasses we had used. Once, she told us: "I enjoy washing the glasses at your grandmother's house because there is a tap in the sink. At home, we have to take them outside and wash them with the water pump or bring water in a bucket to wash them inside when it rains, or it's cold."

We also had friends from downtown. Some of them had new bikes, the latest skates, bags full of marbles, birthday parties with lots of friends, and presents. Others had been to the ocean or had traveled abroad and wore fashionable clothes. It was a completely different reality.

I came to understand humble people in a much deeper way: they had something very different from us. Whether they had little or plenty, they were always grateful for everything that happened around them, for the friends who would listen to them, and the teachers who would teach them how to read and write. Siblings would share everything they had, parents would feed them in the best way they could, neighbors were always ready to help, and animals would provide the milk for the afternoon snack or would keep them company while taking a nap under a tree. They were always grateful and respectful towards life… it was beautiful to spend time with them!

My childhood years, spent between the city and the countryside, hold some of the most rewarding experiences of my life.

My questionnaire kept filling up: how can it be that we are all born with so many differences? Some people lived with comfort, while others could hardly afford to heat their home on chilly days. Some children had large families while other children had no parents; healthy people and sick people; some people had well-paid jobs, while others were looking for work daily to buy food. Some people seemed happy to live this life, while others seemed sad, in pain, and hopeless. And all of them living in the same place.

A vast range of questions opened up to me, and I would become disillusioned just thinking about it. Why hadn't I met anyone yet who shared the same unanswered questions? Why hadn't I received any answers yet?

Some time went by until what would be the start of ten very difficult years for my family and me.

Death knocked at the door time and time again, taking many loved ones without warning, including my aunt, who was the youngest daughter of my beloved grandmother Lucia.

My grandmother's pain was heartbreaking.

Mormons and evangelists would knock at the door with their books and brochures to tell her about God. Sometimes she would listen to them for a few minutes, and sometimes she would thank them and ask them to leave.

Around that time, my mom and dad decided we would move to Buenos Aires. It was such a big change for that young age that I don't remember much of that time. But I do remember when the time came to leave my town. I didn't want to feel that heart-wrenching moment when I had to leave my childhood behind.

It was as if a part of my life was ripped away from me.

We would go back to my town often; the best part was going to visit my grandmother.

Shortly afterward, my grandfather Alberto, my grandmother Lucia's husband and lifelong companion, died; another loss for her and all of us.

He was my beloved "partner-in-crime", one of my teachers, and I was his little princess.

And the following year, my beloved great-grandmother Felicidad left this world at almost 98 years of age.

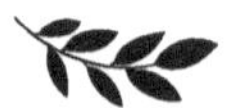

Some years went by and another chapter of my life began to unfold. My grandmother Lucia carried on with her life. It was very hard for her; she would tell every person she encountered about her suffering; she needed answers. She did not understand why so much pain and so many losses over the years... Everything was so different now!

One day as we were going back to Buenos Aires after visiting the town, right before getting in the car, I told her: "Grandma, I'll be back next weekend to see you." She was happy; she was such a beautiful person. Opening her arms as the Portuguese do, she celebrated the fact that I would be returning the following weekend to stay with her for a few days.

That was the last day I saw her. More enlightened, she had accepted and understood what had happened to her daughter, and something bigger made her smile.

My grandmother, my beautiful one. Her mission on this earth had ended.

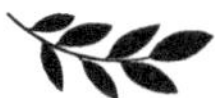

When my grandmother Lucia passed away, my family did not know how to tell Grandma Marina; they loved each other very much, and we did not want the news to affect her. She was older, and we tried to protect her.

I remember the moment when she listened to the news and said: "Lucia was so good, may she rest in peace," with a certainty that it would be so.

She left us all speechless. I came to the conclusion that when people reach a certain age, they understand God and life in a much better way, that perhaps there are no words to describe what we are feeling, or that we may not be prepared to understand it until we reach old age.

I experienced several times what it's like to attend a funeral knowing that the one who left was a loved one, that people come to give you their condolences... It is a void impossible to fill.

I felt the loss of my loved ones like abandonment every time I went back to my town.

I left my heart buried under a tree to be cared for by the animals, butterflies, and summer sunflowers, and I stored my last questions on it: what is the meaning of life and death? Where do we go when we die? Do we no longer exist? What is the purpose of all this? Why so much suffering?

I forgot about my God, that friend who left me here, in this world. It seemed He didn't care whether or not I loved Him. I did not understand why He had taken away what I loved the most in life. I did not understand how He could think I would love Him after allowing so much suffering, how He expected me to love Him with so much pain in my heart. Little by little, I stopped believing in His magnificence; I didn't look at Him anymore; I stopped talking to Him, and I led Him to believe that He had lost me forever.

So many years of unanswered questions, so much pain around me with no explanation.

THE LAST CALL

Two months after we came back to Dubai from the other end of the world, where we had spent a beautiful vacation with our family, I went back to the hospital. This time half of my body was numb.

It seemed as if I had a perfectly drawn line, from head to toe, passing through my navel. One side, both front and back, was numb, and the other half was not.

Back to see my doctor, the nurses, and the MRI machines. What a nightmare!

When they inserted needles into different parts of my body, such as the face, arms, hands, legs, and feet, I did not feel the pricking sensation on the left side. I felt they were inserting something, but it was more like a sensation of electricity running through my body.

Walking was hard; I had lost my balance, and sometimes I had difficulty uttering words. But nobody knew about this.

Back in the MRI room, I thought about asking the technician what he saw in the images. I was hoping he would tell me what I had was not that serious. But when I was inside the scanner with half of my body numb, I thought: "what's happening to me is bad; the images will probably show irreparable damage. Better not to ask. I'd rather not look at his face."

The doctor saw me in his office and showed me in detail the images with the new lesions in my brain and spinal cord.

He confirmed to me that the disease had continued to progress.

My doctor no longer knew what to do with me.

He seemed angry; he couldn't understand why I would not start the drug treatment.

He wrote the name of the drugs again on a piece of paper, and he even told me he would not see me anymore if I didn't realize the risk I was taking. The lapses between episodes were shortening, and the illness was progressing rapidly.

I listened to him and replied: "Thank you, doctor, I'm going to think about it again."

I left the office without looking at him in the eyes. I didn't want to feel the loss of his trust in me. I didn't want to feel what I assumed he was thinking: that I was playing with my health. I didn't want him to believe that I didn't respect him as a doctor. I didn't want him to think that I didn't take his prescription seriously. I didn't want to lose our connection, the only one I had with a healthcare professional.

But indeed, nothing they offered was enough for me.

Perhaps everyone thought I was stubborn and irresponsible, but that was the least of my concerns. I deeply felt I had the right to decide what to do with my body.

After leaving the doctor's office, I went to the emergency room, where they were to start again an intravenous corticosteroid treatment to suppress the inflammation of the nervous tissues.

I was sitting on a stretcher in the nurses' office, and as time went by, I started to feel sick. I was angry, irritated with the whole situation, and while my mind wandered through the places where all the questions of the universe are written, looking for an answer, I had the nurses all over me, squeezing my arms to find a vein where to inject the medication, squeezing me with tubes, and alcohol swabs ... They would insert and remove the needle, and they would reinsert it and remove once again! And at one point, I couldn't take it anymore.

Suddenly, I grabbed the nurse by the arm, pushed her away from me, and started yelling, telling them they didn't know what they were doing.

Why couldn't they find my veins? My arms were hurting from so many needles!

I got up, grabbed my belongings, and stormed out of the hospital.

I ran as much as I could, crying and screaming until I was out of breath. I stopped for a moment and then started walking.

Almost crawling, and with half of my body tingling and swollen, there I was again, like two years ago, walking down the back street of Jumeirah Beach Road.

Everything was the same, but worse.

Reluctantly, I returned to the hospital. Unfortunately, I couldn't go back home like this, with half of my body numb.

I went back into the emergency room with my head down. I assumed everyone had seen what happened; they were waiting for me. Nobody said anything.

For an instant, I thought they must have assumed I was crazy. But I said to myself: "If they already believe I am sick, then for them, I am sick; I suppose it justifies my behavior, doesn't it?"

This time I saw a different nurse whom I knew from before; with the best of intentions and a smile, she handled the entire procedure with utmost care. As she put the dreaded needle in me, I took a deep breath and thanked her.

The loneliness that you feel is impossible to explain. Nobody knows anything about your illness; they take care of you, but they do not know you. They don't understand what is going through your mind or what causes you so much pain, and they don't know how to heal you. They don't know what to say to you nor what to do with you.

In that hospital, I understood that the only thing doctors could offer me were those drugs written on the piece of paper, which I had not looked at, nor was I going to.

For them, I had to follow a drug treatment for life.

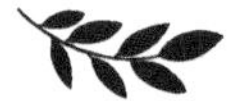

I lived for many years in different places, both in my country and abroad. I believe I have the spirit of my great-grandfather Francisco who dared to cross the ocean several times from Portugal to Argentina. It's the spirit of taking chances, traveling, discovering the treasures that Mother Earth has in every corner of her home, of conquering, of becoming a citizen of the world.

I believe I also carry with me the spirit of my great-grandmother Felicidad: that spirit that always misses its roots, its people, its customs, but adapts, and smiling at life, sows so as to reap its fruits.

Alejandro and I come from different parts of Argentina, just like my great-grandparents in Portugal.

We met in Miami, and like them, shortly after we started dating, we embarked on a new adventure; ours was the "United Arab Emirates."

Whenever I had to move, I did it with an adventurous spirit and full of excitement, but unknowingly, I was reliving a deep silent pain.

I recall when I left Argentina for the first time on the way to Miami, I said goodbye to my family and friends at the airport as if I were going to the town next door. I didn't want to feel the emotions brought on by farewells.

Then a week after arriving at my new home, as I was getting ready to fly to another city in the United States, I felt an intense pain in my back. The pain left me lying on my apartment floor for several hours, unable to move. I had a kidney infection. I couldn't travel.

For many years while living abroad, every time I went back to my village to visit my family, I would get sick with the flu, colds, stomach pain, and fever.

I could see my heart under that tree where I once left it for far too long, without having been aware of it. It was there, alone, with its pain, its memories, its questions, and little by little, as time went by, it hardened.

When we are not whole, and we do not pick up everything we left behind, the body deteriorates.

Life kept testing me more and more; everything regarding my health was becoming more difficult, and I felt I was swimming against the tide: what I was told to do was not what I considered right for me.

I struggled so hard to defend my values and what I considered to be true that I no longer knew who I was.

And there I was, in the United Arab Emirates.

Powerless, exhausted, vulnerable, lost, and unable to find a way out.

GOD'S DAUGHTER

The day came when I dared to look at multiple sclerosis in the eyes and speak to it face to face.

I said: "I created you. It's fine if you stay with me; you are part of me."

And it replied: "I love you, but I want to leave, I'm sorry."

I was puzzled! Where did those words come from?

And that's when I felt like I was dying. Nothing made any sense to me. An erupting volcano from inside of me sparked an explosion with gut-wrenching pain, striking my body and causing me to lose control. My body's tremors made all the locked-up pain I had been secretly carrying all my life shatter like glass.

The unfairness, the abandonment of my loved ones, the uprooting, time and time again.

All the images that make up my life story flashed through my head.

And I cried as I had never cried before. I felt a shock wave so intense that I ended up lying on the ground, in agony, empty and silent.

Yes, I thought I was dying.

As the days went by, unaware I forgot about the deep pain I felt.

I was in a total state of renunciation, surrender, and acceptance.

It was an absolute surrendering of my body, of my being, of everything I had ever been, to life itself.

I surrendered to what was meant to be, to whatever life wanted. In the meantime, I was holding the multiple sclerosis illness gently in my hands, like a lost baby looking for her mother...

We were already two; we were together; we had become close friends.

A few days later, already in better spirits, while playing with Catalina, I saw something that made my eyes open wide; out of the blue, with a big smile on my face, I remembered me, the little girl from the enchanted garden.

I saw myself with my long-sleeved dresses with small flower prints made of a thick winter fabric, with my shoes and socks and my golden curls, surrounded by nature, flowers, bugs, and beings of love. I saw that little girl whose essence lived in connection with her infinite God, the one who cared for her, guided her, forgave her mischiefs, and made her happy.

That God wanted me to remember Him. He had never left me. We had an important agreement, a mission of love to carry out together that had been forgotten. But He was waiting for me.

Remembering that little girl in absolute freedom made my whole being shine. I reached a state where I felt God, my God, deep within my being, and by remembering Him, I realized how much I missed Him.

I asked Him for forgiveness for forgetting Him, and I handed my life over to Him so that He could heal it and we could continue with our mission... Or whatever His will was.

My old identity shed, the one I had created and patched up throughout the years since I had forgotten Him.

I was reborn, or as I used to call it for a long while, I died and woke up while still alive.

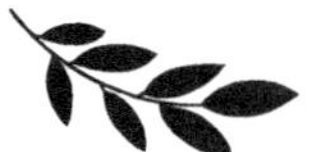

We find God in the depth of our being, beyond the wounds and the weaknesses; in the rubble of the collapsed tower, that tower we build for Him to show Him everything we were able to be and achieve, and how far we were able to go.

We build that tower with few tools or with very fragile tools, somewhat blind, somewhat limping, with a deep longing for love.

That tower cannot stand on its own; it cannot find that blue sky. The staircase does not take us to that place we long for since we first came to this earth.

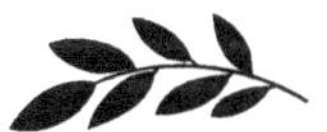

In my dreams, I had a new vision of my reunion with God, which helped me feel Him with more intensity.

In my dreams, God came down to earth, and I got down on my knees before His magnificent and eternal presence. Together, we watched as my entire earthly story fell apart, and through the soul, we looked into each other's eyes and remembered our agreement. With great tenderness and compassion, He extended his hand to me, and I felt completely healed. We both knew that we had to continue what we had planned a long time ago. He helped me stand up, and we melted into an embrace of love.

He is my God.

He and I had decided to HEAL.

Leaving the door open, with nothing in the way, I felt the healing happening together with God. Little by little, my smile reappeared, as did the desire to connect with nature and live life to the fullest.

And now, yes, my illness became my life's best friend.

I accepted it in my life. I embraced it; I thanked it for all the wake-up calls I received; I understood it, came to know it, questioned it so that it would show me how I could set it free; I started loving it the same way I began to love myself, little by little and with compassion.

The energy I felt was different; those were like waves running through my body and moving at a different frequency as if life energy was coming down from the heavens. Everything was in constant movement.

My only priority was to heal myself completely and regain my health.

I was like a saddled horse with blinders on. I had a mission under divine law; there was nothing on my mind except my healing.

My focus, attention, and path were forward.

MY LIFE'S TEACHER

———

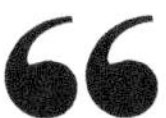

There was someone very significant who was part of my adolescent years and helped shape and give weight to this healing mission that I took upon myself with so much conviction."

Today I am sure that she knew this would happen.

I met Mirna when I was 15 years old. She was a computer science graduate, university professor, historian, astrologer, and flower therapist; a Chinese medicine, anthroposophy and metaphysics student, and a Tao I-chin and Tarot practitioner.

A seer with capital letters! She could see the future of the world, of her patients, the causes of disease, how our body, mind, and spirit worked, and even the most mysterious labyrinths of life.

Mirna lived in her apartment in the "Once" neighborhood in Buenos Aires, Capital Federal.

There you could find the most esoteric and natural information that existed at the time in the entire world: books, writings, research, articles by prestigious doctors, philosophers, archaeologists, objects, graphics, essences, herbs, seeds, some macrame fabric that she made as a meditation practice, and infinite other things. The knowledge you could find in that apartment on Bartolomé Mitre Street was AMAZING.

She took some classes with my mom, and that's how we met.

When I first met her, I asked her to draw my birth chart. After a while, I started going back to her house to learn astrology, and just like that,

I became her student.

With her, I learned about ancient Chinese medicine, the wisdom of our ancestors, the power of medicinal herbs, the path of the soul, that we are energy, that time doesn't exist, and that we came to earth to heal.

Like my grandmothers, she would always tell me: Life is beautiful, Nati!

Whenever she looked at my birth chart, she would tell me that I was coming from the future: that I had to study computer systems analysis; that I had to work with artificial intelligence; that I had to move to Palo Alto, California, that I had to continue studying for the rest of my life, among many other things ... Then she would get lost and continue with comments such as "we must not mutilate the animals anymore; cereals should fill up the fields; not to forget about my country; that we will run out of water." So many things that were foreign to my life back then. At such a young age, it was a challenge to integrate so much information.

But all of it sounded fascinating to me.

Every time I left her apartment, I would take bottles of flower essences with me, among which Walnut* was always a must; it would protect you from hidden enemies.

I would also take jars with blends of medicinal herbs for memory, to eliminate toxins, or to harmonize the body.

She suggested book titles, including naturopathic recipes for the Age of Aquarius, which sometimes we prepared together, plus all the notes on everything we talked about that day ...

Everything esoteric fascinated me, and I spent hours and hours listening to her. Her eloquence seemed to come from another planet.

I loved being by her side with our "mate" for days on end, for many years. She was so magical, so unique, so "herself."

Mirna was a teacher, and for many of us, a medicine woman.

She played an important role in my journey. She served as a guide without me realizing it at the time so that I could reach my longed-for answers in life. But more than anything, she prepared me to stand, or I would rather say, to be firmly rooted at the door of my great mission: healing.

DIVINE GUIDANCE TO THE MAGIC POTION

With a mission in mind and without wasting too much time, I went online to look for information about people who healed themselves of multiple sclerosis. I knew there had to be someone in the world who did.

I found a clinic in China where they practiced Traditional Medicine and treated diseases such as Parkinson's, Epilepsy, Multiple Sclerosis, among others. They recommended in-patient treatment for at least three months.

There was no question in my mind that the clinic could be my first goal. I had nothing to lose. It seemed like a great idea to introduce myself to a group of doctors who think of the body and treat diseases with a different philosophy, and especially a clinic on a mountain in China.

On their page, they reported successful cases of people who healed their illnesses. All the testimonies were there, on the internet.

My husband and the company I worked for, Majid Al Futtaim, supported me in my decision. Their priority was always my health. I just had to organize the trip.

It was amazing how my mind was focusing on nothing but my healing. And of course! When there is a strong intention, everything around it falls into place.

One day around the same time, after taking a different route on the way back home from work, I saw a brown and white sign that said Dubai Herbal Center. I wondered what that could be, and made a U-turn at the roundabout. Today I know that divine guidance led me there.

As I was coming closer to the place, I could not believe what I saw. It was surreal.

I now wonder whether it was real.

It was a white, one-story building in the middle of the desert surrounded by greenery. I left the car under an awning in a parking lot next to the building and walked towards the main entrance under Dubai's scorching sun.

I stood at the front door, unable to see anything inside because of the sun's reflection on the glass. I noticed the sound of the water falling behind me.

When I turned around, I saw a beautiful fountain of fresh and crystalline water. I looked at the plants and flowers around me, and when I looked up, the only thing I saw was sand and more sand...a paradise in the middle of the desert.

I decided to go in!

As the doors opened, I smelled a distinct scent, a unique herbal blend with a refreshing energy. It was definitely a holistic place.

Dubai Herbal and Treatment Center was a holistic medicine center in a desert-like area, founded in 2003 by His Highness General Sheikh Mohammed Bin Rashid Al Maktoum, Vice President of the United Arab Emirates and Sheikh of Dubai.

The Center offered treatments based on Traditional Chinese Medicine, Homeopathy, and Ayurveda.

Without a second thought, I made an appointment right then and there with someone named Dr. María.

I went back home feeling overjoyed.

The day of my appointment at the Dubai Herbal and Treatment Center had come. I arrived early, registered at the reception desk, and a nurse immediately took me to a room to weigh me and take my blood pressure. She then asked me to stay in the waiting room until they called me into the office.

The magazines in the waiting room displayed the colors of nature, advertisements for organic food, articles on how to take care of your body, mind, and spirit, and about how important physical activity, sleep, and rest are.

I was in a place where the philosophy of life was more similar to mine.

They called me, and, to my surprise, the doctor who saw me and the only one at the clinic was Spanish! She was María.

It was such joy to tell a doctor, a woman, what was happening to me, in my own words, in my language. I felt that my words' vibration conveyed much more information about what I was feeling and that she was well aware of that.

In the office with us, next to María, there was a Chinese doctor named Shan Xu.

While I was speaking, she observed me closely and took notes in Chinese in her notebook without understanding a word I was saying.

I was very excited, not only because I was able to express myself, but because they listened and paid close attention to me.

They were with me; they wanted to get to know me, understand me.

I told them about my case, step by step.

I was still taking the corticosteroid medication from the last episode I had.

They asked me to stick my tongue out, and they observed it several times.

The two of them held my hands, one hand each, and they took the three different pulses we have in our wrists. Doctors who practice this type of medicine can feel how your various organs are working through these pulses.

They looked at my eyes, opening them very wide with their fingers. They touched my hands and feet with their hands to feel my body's temperature.

Then they weighed me and took my blood pressure again. The doctor asked me many very interesting questions that no other doctor had ever asked me. For example: What I would usually have for breakfast, lunch, and dinner, at what time, and if I preferred to eat sweet, salty, spicy, or bitter foods. They asked me about my sleep: how many hours I slept, and if I woke up at night; the work I was doing; about my family, my medical history, the color and smell of my urine, how many times a day I had bowel movements, how they looked like, and what color they were; how my period was, what color, if it was regular or irregular, abundant or not; if I did sports, and how many times, and how my body was as a child. They asked me about my state of mind; if I had ever had any trauma or surgery; about my children, if I had ever had a cesarean section; if my hair would fall out; if I was under any medication or if I was taking vitamins; if I perspired; if I preferred to drink warm or cold water, in small sips or not, and how much water a day; whether I felt hot or cold and in what parts of the body, etcetera, etcetera.

With all the answers to those questions and their observations of my body, I felt that these two doctors could understand the condition of my health.

After assessing all the information and reaching a conclusion in her mind, María looked at me and said: "don't worry, we will solve this; we will take care of this; we are going to focus on every area so that we don't leave anything out."

It was like music to my ears. It was the first time someone told me I could heal.

I wondered: could it be that the illness is not as severe as everyone else told me? Did I forget to mention an important detail? Why is she so sure I am going to get better? Is there something magical that everyone is unaware of? Am I dreaming?

I replied: "FINE! Tell me everything I have to do, and I will do it. "

And right there, the Chinese doctor spoke for the first time in English with a Chinese accent and told me: "YOU ARE DRY."

I didn't know what she was referring to until a few years later when I studied Traditional Chinese Medicine, and I understood the big picture of what happened to my body back then: it was totally dry as the Chinese doctor told me, without blood or fluids, without life, dry.

From the office, they took me right away to another room to draw blood for a food intolerance test.

From there, I was taken to another room to have acupuncture. While I was lying down, I remembered the acupuncturist I saw at the very beginning...what a nightmare that day was!

At the end of the tour, they took me to their natural pharmacy, a field which I would study later in life. There, several people were engaged in sifting, cooking, and preparing herbal formulas for the patients.
From the outside, you could smell those magic potions!

Enjoying it and getting used to that distinctive aroma, I waited for my two-liter thermos of tea with an herbal formula prescribed by the Chinese doctor to start my treatment.

Chinese herbs are powerful herbs from nature used for thousands of years to heal the sick, with unique properties that are applied depending on the patient's diagnosis.

These herbs come from leaves, stems, and roots from specific plants born in particular habitats with unique properties to restore the body; there are also parts of some animals, and some minerals.

The combinations of their properties, formulas, and applications first appeared over 5000 years ago in the oldest texts of what we know now as Traditional Chinese Medicine.

Traditional Chinese Medicine looks at the connection among the five elements: water, earth, air, fire, and wood, at the cycles and states of nature, and at the body as a whole to achieve balance and harmony in the body's most natural state.

I went back home with my tea and four big boxes of probiotics and vitamins that came from Germany, and the immense joy and hope that this could be the way.

I ruled out the trip to the clinic in the mountains of China for the time being. I put my trust in María and the Chinese doctor. I trusted the divine guidance that led me to that alternative medicine clinic where they made me feel at home.

Maria was the second push towards my healing.

A few weeks after I started the treatment, they called me to let me know that my food intolerance test results were ready.

I went back to the clinic to find out I was intolerant to gluten, eggs, dairy products, among other substances found in packaged products, and to alcohol.

From that day on, my diet consisted only of meat, fish, fruits, vegetables, legumes, and all kinds of seeds. Water and "mate."

The treatment took one year.

In the beginning, I would go back to the clinic every two weeks. Doctors would do the usual observations, look at my tongue, take the pulses of my wrists to see if they noticed any changes. Depending on how I was doing, they would change and adjust the herbal formula.

I would always leave the clinic with a thermos of freshly prepared warm tea for me, for my body. It felt like a blessing.

I admit I had to get used to the potent smell of the herbs, but over time it became my most delicious magic potion of the day.

After a few months, instead of the herbal tea prepared for me at the clinic, I started taking the herbs in capsules. Those came in bottles, and I had to take them with a glass of water. I kept taking those capsules for years.

The herbs restored my physical body. They helped my body regenerate blood and the various fluids it needed. I needed that oil that makes all corrosion disappear.

They helped my body regenerate tissues, in particular the myelin sheath.

Those herbs knew how to bring the body back to its state of balance and vitality. And that's exactly what they did.

It was one of the best times of my life: I felt I had come back to life.

I had recovered my enchanted childhood garden and had decided to expand it—taking advantage of the opportunity to re-sow the seeds from all those years when I had felt so much pain.

Now, feeling lighter, they would grow stronger, and they would get to see the sun.

THE REFLECTION
OF MY SOUL

_____

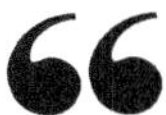

I began to live connected with the cycles of nature, the earth, its energy, its wisdom.

I defied Dubai's heat. I had a garden full of tomatoes and all kinds of green vegetables.

I really enjoyed the beach; I sunbathed and went swimming more than I ever had, in the salty water of the irresistible Persian Gulf.

I started studying everything I found regarding energy, healing, and the esoteric. It had been a long time since I last studied with Mirnuchi (that's how I affectionately used to call Mirna). I was fascinated by all of it. The list was endless.

I connected with my ancestors—my great-grandparents. I looked at their long lives, what they believed in, their thinking, how they lived, and what they ate. I wanted to bring their way of life into mine.

I went to visit an orphanage in the mountain of Khandbari, Nepal, with a friend of mine, a very enriching experience that strongly connected me with my childhood, with service to others, and provided me with plenty of energy to move forward.

The idea of visiting orphanages expanded, with donation visits reaching orphanages in Addis Abas, Ethiopia, including the orphanage of Mother Teresa of Calcutta, Bangalore, India, and Jujuy in Argentina, with lifelong friends.

I cooked and prepared delicious and healthy recipes for everyone.

A South African friend taught me how to bake a delicious, gluten-free, egg-free, dairy-free bread, which turned out to be so delicious and blessed that many called it the blessed bread.

While searching for the miracle of healing, I went to St. Mary's Catholic Church in Dubai where I met Father David.

Father David came from India and was one of St. Mary's Church's priests for many years. One day I went to see him in his office. I will never forget our conversation, and as a token of gratitude for his words, I promised to help him raise funds for the Christian community's Christmas party. I thought about baking the bread I had learned to make and sell it to honor my promise. Everyone liked that bread: it was healthy and delicious. I was sure I could raise something. Not only were we able to help Father David, but we also had several friends who baked this bread for other causes. It was a success; so many people helped and received help. That bread was definitely blessed.

In appreciation, Father David gave me a statue of the Virgin of Fatima. I remember he told me: "Among all the Virgins I have, I felt this is the one that you should take home with you."

The Virgin of Fatima is the Virgin Mary who appeared to the three shepherd children in Fátima, Portugal, my great-grandparents' home country.

I discovered the beauty of Dubai! Every day, I fell more in love with its people, culture, beliefs, way of life, and buildings!

I promised myself I would show my children how beautiful life is.

The moment had come when I understood my grandmother Marina's words: "Life is beautiful, baby."

Yes, Grandma!

It never crossed my mind during that time to wonder whether I was healing or how the lesions were doing. I knew what was happening; I could feel it in the depth of my being: I was healing, healing my being, recovering the "Nati" that I had forgotten. I knew how to do it.

Whenever I go over my history, its characters, traits, words, places, and my words and thoughts… I clearly see that everything reflected my soul. Indeed, what we see every second of our lives is a reflection of our soul, neither bad nor good; it's neutral; it can be good or bad depending on how we want to look at it.

Everything around us is a projection of our inner world.

Now I can see the fire burning inside me and drying up my body, consuming my blood, fluids, and even my myelin sheath. It was the same fire I felt those days walking under the blazing sun on Jumeirah Beach Road.

Now I look at the MRI machine's confinement as my encapsulated pain, wanting to break free.

Now I see the nurse poking me with the needle, again and again, trying to find my vein: it was my anger looking for a door to escape.

I had so many emotions in turmoil, so much pain, anger, so many questions, and above all, I had lost my connection with divine energy, the energy that created us!

I needed that energy—the fuel that keeps us alive, nourishes, and protects us—to flow from the source into my body. That energy comes from Heaven and Earth, and I had to make room and space for it to enter my body.

I had been angry, always resisting the greatest thing that exists: The

Almighty, the Omnipotent, and the Omnipresent. I had turned my back on Him as I had never turned my back on anyone. And this had set my body and my soul on fire.

My heart had become so hardened that the doors to God had closed.

I can see now that I had to take just one step, but how difficult it is to see it and feel it!

That step was to accept those ten years of pain, hold them tight and let them go, let them fly until they reached the light. That step was to understand that everything in life is born, dies, and transforms itself; that everything changes, and the more we resist what is happening to us, the greater the suffering and the more it expands like a grey cloud, while our essence fades away.

That step was to recover my heart.

Pain needs us; it requires us to take it out of the dark and gloomy dungeon where it doesn't see the light, and where the wound keeps bleeding more and more.

Our pain is crying out for us to remember it, to remember that it is part of us.

Our pain wants us to acknowledge it, accept it, forgive it and guide it into the light.

By looking at it with compassion, it will grow wings and fly towards the light.

And the reflection of our soul will change at that very instant.

When we have the courage to take these steps, we are reborn time and again, and we feel like butterflies, light, beautiful, transformed.

We have to accept with our whole being that what happened or is happening to us is perfect and necessary for us: there are no culprits, nothing, and no one.

It is all about an agreement between you and God.

BETWEEN HEAVEN
AND EARTH

It was my birthday. It was almost a year since my ongoing treatment with Traditional Chinese Medicine had started. Once I started the treatment, I experienced no more episodes of multiple sclerosis.

That morning, while having breakfast, I felt the desire to honor the changes that were taking place in my body and felt the urge to celebrate and follow up with it.

Right then and there, I called the Neuro Spinal Hospital and made an appointment for an MRI of my brain and spinal cord.

I wanted to know what my body looked like inside and find out if there was anything else that I could do to help this transformation.

That evening I celebrated my birthday with friends at the PF Chang restaurant in Emirates Mall. We reserved a table in a secluded area used for special occasions.

I remember that as a starter, it was customary to order Dynamite Shrimps for everyone; I was certainly tempted, but I stuck to my strict diet. I hadn't missed a single day. Besides, I had a favorite dish: Beef a La Sichuan. With that, I was happy.

During dinner, I told my friends that I was going to have an MRI done the following week to check how my body was doing. To this day I remember that moment; everyone told me that I had already healed.

But I didn't say anything; I wanted to wait to see the results.

And the day came! When we entered the hospital with Alejandro, I felt like a new person.

The place was the same, and many things had not changed: the scent of the reception area; the silence of the people sitting in the waiting room; the sound of the coffeemaker in the cafeteria located at the center of the building, and the reflection of the sun entering through its only windows in the ceiling; the few potted plants placed in different sections, and the cold temperature of the building, so that I always had a coat with me.

But time had passed, and I no longer belonged to that place. I knew I was just visiting.

While in the waiting room, I observed many young Arab women covered with their black abayas*, sitting, waiting to see a doctor. I wondered if they were multiple sclerosis patients since the hospital specialized in neurological issues.

I fantasized about talking with them about the treatment I was undergoing but doubted they would be interested.

I thought it was odd that it wasn't an option for the Emirati people. The Sheik of Dubai, much loved by his community, was after all the founder of the alternative medicine clinic Dubai Herbal and Treatment Center, where I was being treated with traditional Chinese medicine by María, a Western and Eastern medical doctor.

Of course, some Emirati people attended that alternative medicine clinic. However, not as many as the number of patients in this waiting room. And who knows how many more there were in the city.

"What was holding people back? Why don't they trust thousand-year-old medicine? Do they know about it? What drives people to inject themselves with drugs for life?" Those were my thoughts as I waited my turn for the MRI procedure that I was about to undergo for the first time without experiencing any symptoms.

I heard my name being called. I got up and followed a nurse who went with me to the room where I would have the procedure done.

This time, while lying down on the MRI machine, I spoke to my body and thanked it for allowing this procedure one more time.

I hugged it; we closed our eyes, and with an eternal smile, together we set the intention that this would be the last time.

The doctor welcomed me in his office after almost a year from the time he last saw me. He already had the results. He sat down at his desk, opened the computer to show us the images, and smiled at me. There were no new lesions in either the spinal cord or the brain. And in the upper area of the cervical cord, the three lesions that were there before had entirely disappeared.

How amazing my dear magical herbs had been! Alejandro and I exchanged a complicit look. He always knew that I would heal.

In the report, for the missing lesions, the doctor used the phrase "completely resolved."

Overjoyed, I asked my doctor: "Aren't you going to ask me what I'm doing?"

He didn't say anything; he just smiled. I told him everything. He listened to me paying close attention.

Then he asked me to wait for him for just a moment.

He left the office and returned with the clinic director and the other doctor whom I had seen only twice before. Those were the three Iraqi doctors, the same ones who came to visit me when I was initially hospitalized.

While they talked and discussed in Arabic, checking the images and my medical history, I just observed the situation, saw their astonished faces, and listened to them, feeling so happy, finding it impossible to hide the giant smile on my face...

At that very moment, I declared myself completely HEALTHY AND HAPPY.

I had a brand-new body thanks to Traditional Chinese Medicine ...

My mind was transformed thanks to my persistent intention to heal myself and regain my vitality.

My spirit was transformed thanks to my reconnection with God and His divine guidance.

My spiritual, mental, and physical bodies, in that exact order, reached a state of harmony.

For everyone, it was a miracle.

And why not believe that perhaps we can perform miracles on our own?

SACRED
TREASURE

*Through the experience of illness
and healing, I received an invaluable
treasure.*

A treasure that came through my heart with divine knowledge and
helped me restore my spirit, mind, and body.

A treasure full of pearls that pour like rainfall whenever I need guidance.

It was a treasure that opened the doors of my heart and allowed those
existential questions I had as a child to reveal some answers.

Those answers came to me from several sources and in different
shapes and nuances—it was like putting together a big puzzle of infinite
possibilities.

The mystery inherent in the answers to our existential questions is not
supposed to reveal itself easily. It requires that we immerse ourselves
with all our being into the unknown, into a fresh new way of looking at
reality.

This chapter is about that—about that little girl who found her treasure.
In her own words, she will tell you the most sacred teachings that we
discovered together on this healing journey.

OUR
PRECIOUS GIFT

Coming to Earth is a precious gift; what we, as souls, desire the most is to come here to contribute to the transformation of our consciousness. It is all part of a divine plan of which we are all part, and it has to do with LOVE.

We could all experience what unconditional, genuine love, is; we have felt it intensely in the arms of God, which is the place where we belong.

That place that some have called heaven, in that place we are all one, we don't have a body; we are like light dancing; we are lightweight, without baggage, feeling great joy, bathed in eternal love, unlimited happiness, an explosion where all the parts spread out and find a place where they all fit, all intertwined: we are all there, and it feels so good; that is our home, the Kingdom of God, divine consciousness.

Part of the divine plan is to search for the parts of our consciousness that got lost and are not vibrating at the level of love. Love is the highest vibration that keeps us all together and at home.

Our souls are the ones helping with this plan; we came to Earth with a specific mission agreed upon before our arrival.

We are like worker bees working for the queen, with a common divine plan, and we will not stop until we achieve it: that information is engraved in our BEING.

OUR
BIG SECRET

When we come to Earth, we forget where we come from and what we came here to do. It happens this way because that's how we can profoundly learn from life experiences.

We come here carrying a suitcase with tools, a consciousness to transform, and specific tasks for this purpose.

Think of low-vibration consciousness as smoke, which we see when we burn something; that smoke is grey or black.

Think of high vibration consciousness as bright light, with movement and vibrant colors. It would be like looking through a kaleidoscope of infinite perfect geometric figures dancing and shining, but at maximum power.

We are like light bulbs that can be turned on or off depending on the consciousness level surrounding us.

Lower vibration consciousness transforms itself into higher frequency consciousness when we pass the lessons we came here to learn. We must go through the pain, feel it, embrace it, forgive it, accept it, transform it, and ultimately transcend it.

That is how the smoke will transform into colored sparks, and darkness will transform into light.

Little by little and incessantly, we will receive more and more light, and we will get a chance to remember who we are.

Our great secret is to forget so that we can remember.

OUR EARTH

When we open our eyes and look around, we see so much magnificence that, for a moment, we become speechless.

A limitless sky, stars that shine at unreachable distances, seeds born, flowers that bloom, birds that fly, immense oceans that are home to underwater worlds that we have not yet fully discovered.

The sun that is here every day, the spectacular moon, the energy of the planets in our Solar System, their movements, the mountains, the forests, the jungles, and the beautiful animal species all inhabiting the same place.

We must be very important to be part of this magnificence! Have you ever wondered about that?

How can one not wonder who we are, what we are doing in this world, where we came from, and where we are going?

So many existential questions that we hardly ask ourselves, and that we ignore because no one can give us answers we can comprehend.

And we stop asking ourselves those questions because our glorious mission requires that we do not get to that information. It requires concentration on what we came here to do; therefore, these questions are always pending, but one day we will get to know the answers... on Earth or in the afterlife.

OUR PLAN
IS PERFECT

We are perfectly designed so that our plan unfolds according to what we agreed before coming here.

We choose our parents, our place of birth, even the day and time to receive the energy required from the planets at that specific moment in time.

The map of the heavens at the precise moment we were born is engraved in our cells.

It is a perfect plan energetically designed for each day of our lives.

We have agreements with other souls as well that will help us in our learning. Some will love us, others will teach us something important for our life, and others will leave us. Thanks to them, we can advance our learning.

And we are also teachers of other souls. We are all teachers and learners. Or maybe we are our own teachers and learners.

Usually, the first part of our lives is meant to prepare us for the plan we brought in with us.

We are born with a vast amount of light, reflected in our eyes' brightness, but as the months and years go by, that light fades away.

We don't find that unconditional love that we knew before; what we receive does not fulfill us; it confuses us; it saddens us. And we believe we are not enough.

Somehow, we learn how to live in a society on Earth. We learn to comply with rules and mandates, experiment without having prior information, believe what we hear, and memorize. We learn to desire, make mistakes, humiliate ourselves, cry, challenge ourselves, fall, get up, wish, suffer, change directions, understand, love again, forget, forgive, and let go.

We create our personality, our mask, which hides who we really are. We hold on to certain beliefs, and our ego defends us from any attack on what we think we are.

We go through painful situations, sometimes traumatic, and we store them in our suitcases.

We become so disconnected from everything that, at some point, we can only rely on ourselves. We don't want to get hurt anymore. We don't want to experience more pain, and we create a shell with one sole purpose: not to feel anymore.

We forget what happened to us; we don't want to look at it; sometimes we are ashamed of it; it makes us feel vulnerable. We think it belongs to the past, and we minimize it. We hide it and don't want "what happened" to us to define us.

OUR BAGGAGE

And there we go walking through life, carrying a suitcase full of experiences on our back, with a low-frequency consciousness to transform, ours and our ancestors.

That consciousness has a mechanism, and it is crucial to understand it: it attracts situations to our life of a similar frequency for us to see them. Through the process of feeling and understanding, we can transform them and transcend them.

To recognize them, those will be the situations that do not bring us peace. Unfortunately, we often run away from them; we get angry; we defend ourselves.

Often, we do not allow "that thing" that we are feeling to be recognized by us, to be seen and observed.

And that is how the suitcase becomes heavier and heavier.

Those situations that don't bring us peace rob us of our freedom, joy, enjoyment, and happiness.

With time the physical, mental, and spiritual bodies deteriorate. The smoke expands and does not let in the light that nourishes us and regenerates us. That light is our essence.

And that's when, most of the time, illnesses manifest in the physical body.

There may be other ways that the diseases that we know of develop, but this is one of them.

Thank goodness the day comes when our soul puts the suitcase down, opens it little by little, and transforms the caterpillars inside into butterflies so they can fly.

This process is about opening our eyes then dare to see what is inside that suitcase, feel whatever is there, connect with that painful situation, with the emotions, feel them in the body, contemplating them while they last, not attempting to block them, but embracing them. It is about remembering that they are ours, that they have been there with us for a long time, and that they only want to transform themselves into sparks of color.

It is time for us to set them free, to dare to be vulnerable, to trust in what we came here to do: to develop our consciousness and harvest the royal jelly from heaven.

Use this magical moment to become a fairy or a wizard and watch the magic you can make using this divine formula.

The faster we go through this process, the faster suffering will fade away, inner peace will flourish, and the happier we will walk through life.

We will find many answers in our past, but the key to opening the path to our soul's salvation lies inside of us.

Picture yourself above you, and from there, look at yourself. What do you see? What do you hear? What do you feel when you observe?

What you perceive at every instant since you were born reflects your inner world so that you can see it. What you dislike or makes you feel uncomfortable is there to show you there is something you must transform. What you love is also part of you; it is that force, that divine light that is always with you.

What we see, what they do to us, what they tell us, what enters us through all our senses, the disease itself is us talking to ourselves. It is the reflection of our consciousness at that very moment.

What you believe your reality to be, is a perfect mirror, just for you.

OUR BELIEFS

Part of the healing formula is to examine our beliefs. What do we believe in? What do we believe to be possible or impossible?

The belief that I was a healthy person and that I could never get sick made me resist what was happening. I could not accept in any way that I was ill.

This attitude made my body deteriorate more every day, and my days of suffering became more intense. Everything became more pronounced, sped up, and overflowed, thus delaying the healing process.

Until the day came when I accepted it.

But because of my conviction: "I don't believe that God designed our bodies to be able to get sick without being able to heal," the search for the permanent healing of my body became my sole priority, and I was able to find it only when I became one with Him. Of course, He had to tell me where to look to find it.

It is crucial to challenge what is "true" in our beliefs. Being honest with the ideas that do not serve us and having the courage to change them is a valuable exercise for transformation.

OUR MEDICINE

Nature possesses the medicine that heals human beings.

Its energy is pure, it connects to heaven and earth, and that is the energy we need to return to our most pristine state.

We must connect in the same way trees do, with our feet on mother earth and looking up at the stars.

We must connect with mother earth because our bodies are from the earth; only she knows what medicine will nourish us and regenerate us. Her consciousness codes are the key to restoring our physical body until the day comes when we return this incredible body to her, this sacred temple that we borrowed from her.

We must connect with the stars, because our soul is eternal and belongs to the divine consciousness, to the universe.

Without heaven and earth, it would be difficult for us to experience our divine right to enjoy life to the fullest.

Our medicine comes from heaven and earth.

OUR REALITY

What we imagine, think, say, and feel ... we actually CREATE.

When they told me: "you have multiple sclerosis, it's a disease that for the time being has no cure,"... something inside me stopped listening because I knew at a subconscious level that what we imagine and feel manifests itself. And if I continued to listen and pay attention, I was going to believe what the doctors were telling me. If I thought about it in the way it was being conveyed to me (with fear, concern, hopelessness), THAT would be my reality at that moment.

From day one, I did not want that reality in my life.

One of the gifts I brought with me to this earth is the gift of keeping my mind blank in situations that have a low-frequency vibration, in those circumstances that are not the best for me. It is instantaneous; I pause when I detect something that is not in harmony with what I want in my life.

My blank mind does not think about anything, does not judge, does not analyze, does not imagine, does not change words; it remains silent.

That silence keeps my life flowing, without ties or conditions, fully trusting that "what is"—is right at that moment.

That space, that emptiness, gives me the strength to wait for the time when I can focus on the thoughts that I desire, those of a higher vibration, of a higher frequency, beautiful thoughts.

Focusing on the thoughts of the highest vibration is the most valuable exercise we can ever learn. Those should be thoughts in harmony with the divine, with the miraculous, so that they can manifest in our reality.

I knew that being ill would be temporary because it was not the vibration coherent with my deepest desires.

Realities are temporary; we can change our life just by imagining and feeling what we imagine. We are creators—a great responsibility.

Sometimes we don't take the time to examine what we want for ourselves.

Do we know what we want? And when we do, do we believe it's possible?

It is crucial to have a clear intention of what you want: if the purpose is true healing, recovering your vitality, your health, your life ... then trust, have faith, and ask for help without fear. What difference does it make! Nothing to lose.

What happens to you is perfect, and you can be sure that you have an army of heavenly beings around you waiting for you to ask them to be by your side, to guide you, to show you the road you have to travel.

Once you are sure of what your desire is and when you come to imagine it, visualize it and feel it fulfilled in all its splendor, the last magic touch that will help manifest it will be to feel, from the bottom of your heart, that you can also live without your wish being fulfilled.

When you can truly live with that desire or without it, with illness or without illness, and you allow it to be the will of God or the universe, they will easily grant you your wish.

You will have released what you want and what you don't want, what you think you should or shouldn't, what you think you deserve and don't deserve, what you think you are and you are not.

When you are on good terms with what is, with what life gives you, with what life shows you, and you give thanks for it with joy, your desire will manifest.

These manifestations we sometimes call them miracles.

We are a miracle, and the day will come when we will know we can perform miracles.

Our ultimate goal in everything we experience is to embrace the whole, the good and the bad, the light and the dark, the cherished yin yang.

To embrace the divine plan agreed upon before coming to Earth.

OUR PURPOSE

We go through many situations and experiences in life. All of it has a purpose which we have forgotten since we first arrived here: to love ourselves again.

Our primary job here is first to learn how to love ourselves again. We can achieve this through inner work.

Transforming our consciousness is the path towards LOVE.

Our path is up to us; incidents will occur, but it's only up to us to look at them with acceptance and reverence. We will all arrive at the same destination; it is up to us which way to take.

And then, we will be able to love our neighbor, but first, we have to love ourselves.

"Love your neighbor as yourself"; when you love yourself, you will love your neighbor.

Our purpose is to love ourselves again.

OUR PATH

One day I understood that life is about looking at yourself.

One day I understood that to heal is to love oneself again.

One day I understood that illness is a lesson that we teach ourselves to help us remember who we are.

Together with God, who is within us, we are the only ones who possess the truth and know the path to healing. Only with Him we can plan what we want to do to heal our souls.

There is deep meaning in a person's experience with illness; it is so sacred that we can't comprehend it unless we go through it.

How brave are those souls who decide to go through a disease to remember what we all forget, what we all long for, remembering where we come from! Remember who we are!

How brave! What an amazing healing mission it is to decide to love yourself again and love everything with compassion.

Remembering will be the greatest blessing you have ever imagined; it will be a miracle.

Open your horizons; they are infinite...

Open your heart, even if it hurts ...

Open your mind, even if it's sealed ...

Open yourself to new possibilities, make the impossible possible.

Challenge yourself; dare to live!

Venture to imagine, like a child, and without limitations the reality you want for your life, with your arms open to the entire universe, and with the right to live to the fullest, as you have always wanted, playing and experiencing every second of your life.

Start by taking off your shoes and walking barefoot on the ground; feel the energy of the earth.

And the first night you see the sky full of stars have a conversation with them.

They are waiting for you; connect with the heavens because we are made of that same energy, and their energy will help you restore yours.

It is my deepest wish that you find the magic that you carry within, and that everything around you lights up like the BRIGHTEST star in the entire UNIVERSE.

I now know that our path is to return to God and that illness is an opportunity to accomplish that.

Thank you for being you.

YOU ARE UNIQUE,
AND YOU HAVE
AN AGREEMENT
<u>WITH</u> GOD

I would like you to know that you are unique and you have an agreement with God.

That life is a unique opportunity to be enjoyed and not wasted, and that pain is part of our salvation.

We are not who we think we are; we aren't anything nor anyone; we are light, a spark of light that is all and nothing at the same time: this is who we are.

We have believed a thousand things; we have held on to the idea that we are who we think we are. And we hold on to it.

And even if we are not to blame, that is our misfortune; that misfortune makes us suffer more than we should.

We have forgotten who we are, and it is a challenge to remember.

We have many layers of limitations that weaken us, that don't let us be free. The only thing left for us is to learn how to remove those layers, one by one, incessantly.

And to remember that we have guidance every step of the way to help us find the thread that will unravel our old, tangled, and wounded ball of yarn that doesn't let us fly.

There are thorns and holes along our path, but once we know the destination is that which we planned together with God, the wounds from those thorns will strengthen us, and from rock bottom, we will see the light of God.

Because the agreement we have with Him is divine; it is an absolute beauty; it is fulfillment; it is salvation.

And that's where we are all going, all of us together, in unity, in communion.

SPECIAL: MAY YOUR BODY BE A SANCTUARY!

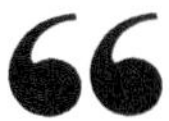

The most important aspect in the healing process is your connection with the spiritual world, with divine energy, with whatever you think that is, the greatest thing there is.

With those magnificent beings and energy that surround us, some forms invisible to most people's eyes: archangels, angels, guides, ancestors, virgins, saints, spiritual teachers, nature, stars, crystals, sacred objects, that which resonates with you, with that most intimate and sacred part of you, they will be your divine guidance.

Look for something that resonates with you and makes your heart expand when you have it in front of you.

That is how you can receive answers to your questions. You will start hearing what they want to tell you and you will be able to talk, understand, laugh with them and find the meaning to many things that now have no explanation for you.

To succeed at this, something powerful that I learned in the past few years is to create an altar, your own altar in a corner of your home.

In the sacred place that you create following your intuition, you can have whatever makes you feel connected with the spiritual world at that moment in time.

For the last few years, for example, I had placed on my altar the Virgin of Fátima that Father David gave me, which meant a lot to me. I also had a little elephant, a representation of Ganesh from India, a present from a very dear friend of mine, and some angels I was very fond of that I bought during a crystal healing course. My beloved Jesus, my dear Buddha, a mandala that I bought on my trip to Nepal, which connects me with sacred geometry, a rosary of the Virgin of Guadalupe, a golden toad representing my fears, some crystals, leaves of a tree, water, and many other things.

Your altar may have a photo of a relative who is no longer here and a candle; this will be more than enough to connect with divine energy.

Once your altar is set up, you'll have a spot for when you need to communicate with your guides. They know more than anyone else what you need, and the step you have to take towards healing.

When you are ready, you may sit in front of the altar, light a candle, and with your eyes closed, visualize this: intending to heal, call on the Creator of Heaven and Earth, the father universe, and our beloved mother earth. Feel their love for you and return that love to them. Visualize that you embrace them with all your heart. Call upon the angels, archangels, your personal guides, all the teachers and beings in front of you, and, through your sacred space, ask for protection, guidance, and healing.

Once you have called everyone and felt their energy, you can say: "the altar is open." Everything in front of you will be inside you; the reflection of your soul is always with you.

This precious moment is sacred to you. In that space, you can speak, ask, and listen; everything that goes through your mind is a conversation between you and everything beyond; learn to listen, feel, and trust the words that come through all your senses.

Be patient, wait, have faith and trust.

It is important to write down the information that you receive. You can do it while you are there.

Feel as if you were talking to people you have always known.

Feel comfortable; they know the innermost depths of your soul. Enjoy this moment; whatever you want to do, do it: it is your date with the spiritual world.

And the most beautiful thing is that you can do it as many times as you want and for as long as you want.

When you're done, give thanks to everyone for their presence, protection, guidance, and healing with all your heart. Give thanks, give thanks, give thanks.

The day will come when you will converse with them all the time. That will be when your body becomes a sanctuary, and divine guidance will be part of your life.

Light up your altar, shine your light…

And so be it!

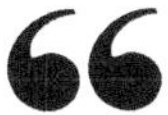

There comes a time when you understand everything, but there are no words to describe it, and very few will listen to you.

There comes a time when you know more every day, and at the same time, you don't know anything. You know less every day.

There comes a time when life is beautiful, and at the same time you know it´s not real.

There comes a time when you know you are not from this earth, that you are just passing by, and the only thing that matters to you is to heal what you have come here to heal.

ACKNOWLEDGMENTS

Especially, and with all my love to Alejandro, my beloved life partner, who knows me better than anyone else. I am wholeheartedly thankful for his presence.

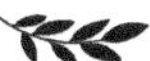

To our beloved children, Catalina, and Jerónimo, for reminding us every day what life is all about.

To my parents and siblings, whom I love with all my heart: Aldo, Mabel, Marianela, and Hernán, for silently supporting me and fully trusting me at all times.

In loving memory of my grandmother Lucía, my grandmother Marina and my teacher Mirna, three stars shining through all eternity, for showing me how beautiful life is.

To all those who were by my side during the healing of my illness. Especially Dr. María Ridao Alonso, the Dubai Herbal and Treatment Center team, the Neuro Spinal Hospital team, and the support represented by Majid Al Futtaim

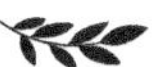

To those friends that God put on my path to inspire me to write this story: Daniela Martinez Vertiz, Justine Martin, Suzanne Gidwani; and Yana Murguía, who devoted her divine energy to make this publication a success.

GLOSSARY

Abaya is a simple and loose-fitting dress, similar to a robe, worn by women in some parts of the Muslim world. The traditional abaya is black and covers the entire body except for the head, feet, and hands. Women also wear a scarf to cover the head and shoulders; some women wear the nicab, a facial veil that covers everything but the eyes.

Al Safa is a residential area in Dubai, known as home to one of the city's largest lungs, a vast park (Al Safa Park), full of trees, where people can enjoy the outdoors.

Allah is the Arabic word used to refer to God in the Islamic religion.

Multiple sclerosis is a disease of the brain and spinal cord (central nervous system). It damages the myelin sheath, the substance that surrounds and protects nerve cells. This damage slows down or blocks messages between the brain and the body, leading to multiple sclerosis symptoms. These can include vision disorders, muscle weakness, sensory changes, paralysis, tingling, problems with coordination and balance, phenomena such as numbness, itching or pricking, difficulties with thinking and memory, among others.

If the disease continues to progress, people lose the ability to write, see, speak, or walk.

Majid Al Futtaim is an Emirati business executive, founder, owner, and president of the Majid Al Futtaim Group.

Mam o Ma'am is another written form for Madam (lady) that people use to address a woman politely or respectfully. Mam is a distorted form of the word Madam.

Mate is an infusion of dried and ground yerba mate leaves, served in a container of the same name and into which is poured boiling water, making "mate" or, if we use cold water, "tereré." We drink it through a metal straw [bombilla]. The container is for group use; it is not usually used individually unless drinking the infusion by yourself. Customs vary slightly by region, but in most South American countries they agree on sharing the container and the metal straw.

Ramadan is the ninth month of the Islamic calendar, respected by Muslims worldwide as the month of fasting, prayer, reflection, and community. It is a celebration of Muhammad's first revelation. Fasts run from sunrise to sunset. People work fewer hours during the day; food places close until dusk, and, with a few exceptions, it is forbidden for non-Muslims to eat, drink, smoke, chew gum in public.

Walnut is the flower used to protect against external influences and the effects of a particular change. Bach Walnut Flower Essence helps break the bond with the past and release ties to move forward with confidence and without unnecessary suffering.

BIBLIOGRAPHY

Bibliography suggested by the author for transformation and healing

Anselm Grün & Meinrad Dufner: Health as a spiritual task.
Barbara Ann Brennan: Hands of Light; A guide to healing through the Human Energy Field.
Barbara Ann Brennan: Light Emerging; The journey of personal healing.
Brian Brownie Walker: El Tao I-Chin de Lao Tzu.
David R. Hawkins: Healing and Recovery.
Drunvalo Melchizedek: Living in The Hearth.
Eva Pierrakos & Donovan Thesenga: Surrender to God within.
Eva Pierrakos: The Pathwork of Self-transformation.
Foundation for Inner Peace: A Course in Miracles.
Gonzalo Rodriguez-Fraile: A new paradigm of reality?.
Louise Hay: You can heal your life.
Lynne Paige Walker & Ellen Hodgson Brown: Natures Pharmacy: Break the Drug Cycle With Safe Natural Alternative Treatments for 200 Everyday Ailments.
Marianne Williamson: A Return to Love.
Paul U. Unschuld & Hermann Tessenow: Huang Di Nei Jing Su Wen: A foundation of Chinese life sciences and medicine.
San Agustín:The City of God.
Susan Thesenga: The Undefended Self: Living the Pathwork
Taylor Caldwell: Dear and Glorious Physician: A Novel about Saint Luke.
Ted J. Kaptchuk: The web that has no weaver, Understanding Chinese Medicine.
Thorwald Dethlefsen & Rudiger Dahle: The Healing Power of Illness.

ABOUT THE AUTHOR

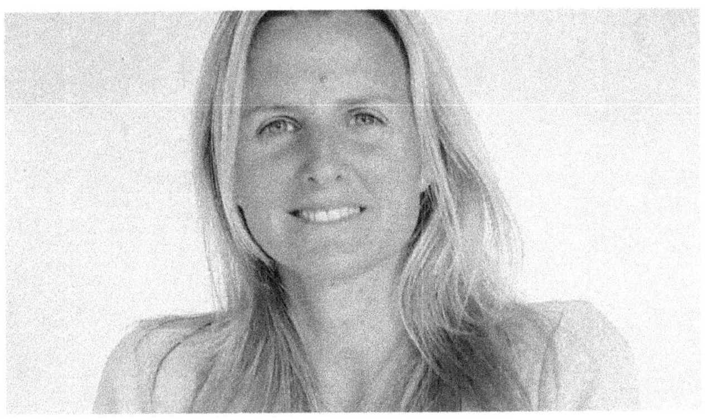

Natalia Orsi is originally from Argentina, currently living with her family in Miami, USA.

She has dedicated her life to her two big passions. First, the evolution of technology, with over 20 years dedicated to her professional career and the innate ability to contribute unconventional ideas, leading her to successful jobs with companies in Latin America, the United States, and the Middle East.

And her main passion has been the evolution, existence, and behavior of humanity, nature, planet Earth, the entire universe, and the connection among all of them. The existential questions she had since an early age, and her interest in the esoteric world, the unknown, and the great truths that lie behind our existence have been the engine that led Natalia to discover the secret to her healing and to understand a little better what our passage through life really means.

This book was completed in August 2020. Natalia didn't have any more lesions, and the Multiple Sclerosis illness completely disappeared.